Chaker JABER
Imene MAGROUN
Nadia MOULAHI Abir AYADI

Arteriovenous fistulas

Chaker JABER
Imene MAGROUN
Nadia MOULAHI Abir AYADI

Arteriovenous fistulas

Creation of arteriovenous fistulas for endovascular hemodialysis: A review of the literature

ScienciaScripts

Imprint

Any brand names and product names mentioned in this book are subject to trademark, brand or patent protection and are trademarks or registered trademarks of their respective holders. The use of brand names, product names, common names, trade names, product descriptions etc. even without a particular marking in this work is in no way to be construed to mean that such names may be regarded as unrestricted in respect of trademark and brand protection legislation and could thus be used by anyone.

Cover image: www.ingimage.com

This book is a translation from the original published under ISBN 978-620-3-43982-3.

Publisher:
Sciencia Scripts
is a trademark of
Dodo Books Indian Ocean Ltd. and OmniScriptum S.R.L Publishing group
Str. Armeneasca 28/1, office 1, Chisinau-2012, Republic of Moldova, Europe
Printed at: see last page
ISBN: 978-620-5-28512-1

Creation of arteriovenous fistulas for endovascular haemodialysis: A review of the literature

Table of contents

Introduction

Chronic kidney disease is the progressive loss of kidney function. It is defined, independently of its cause, by the presence of markers of kidney damage or a drop in the glomerular filtration rate (GFR) calculated below 60 ml/min/1.73 m^2 body surface area for more than three months. GFR is used to classify patients into five stages of renal failure, the last of which is end-stage renal disease (ESRD) defined by a GFR below 15 ml/min/1.73 m [2](1).

In CKD, renal replacement is essential in the short term to sustain life. Haemodialysis (HD) is the most common modality of renal replacement for patients with CKD. Millions of people worldwide are on HD (1). In Tunisia, an estimated 9,500 kidney patients at the stage of CKD are on HD (2).

This method of extra-renal purification requires access to blood via a peripheral vascular approach. The success of this vascular approach depends essentially on the pre-operative assessment, which must systematically include an interrogation, a meticulous clinical examination, arterial and venous Doppler ultrasound of the upper limbs and, if necessary, phlebography or a phleboscanner (3).

The ideal vascular approach must meet several essential criteria (1) including :

-	provide a minimum blood flow of 600 ml/min,

-	be sustainable (used several times a week for long periods),

-	have minimal risk of thrombosis and infection, and

-	suitable for the patient.

Several types of vascular access have been developed to meet these different criteria to a greater or lesser extent. They are generally classified into three categories:

- native arteriovenous fistulas (AVFs),

- arteriovenous bypass surgery and

- HD catheters, whether temporary or permanent (3).

Native AVF is considered to be the best vascular approach. Prosthetic arteriovenous bypass grafts, indicated when a native approach is not possible, are more prone to complications, especially infectious ones. Central venous catheters, indicated in the emergency setting, are a standby solution but are frequently complicated by serious infections and central venous stenosis which threaten future vascular approaches. (4).

Recently, new minimally invasive techniques for endovascular AVF fabrication have emerged: the Ellipsys® system and the WavelinQ™ system. The Ellipsys® System is a single catheter venous access system using thermal energy that allows the creation of an arteriovenous anastomosis by tissue fusion between the proximal radial artery (PRA) and the adjacent perforating vein of the elbow (PVO). The WavelinQ™ system is a dual catheter venous access system carrying magnets and an electrode transmitting electrical current from a radiofrequency (RF) generator that creates communication between the radial or ulnar artery and their satellite deep vein (5).

The objective of this literature review was to evaluate the efficacy and safety of endovascular AVF creation systems in patients with ESRD.

Methods

Presentation of the work

In this work, we conducted a review of the literature with a view to identifying the place of endovascular techniques in the creation of blood access. The native AVF created by surgery is, until now, the gold standard. The objective of this work was to evaluate the efficacy and safety of endovascular AVF creation systems in patients with ESRD.

Bibliographic research

We conducted a literature search using the following search engines "PubMed", "Google Scholar", "Science Direct" and "Cochrane Library" from the first publication date in January 2015 until May 2021 to identify all published articles related to our research topic.

www.pubmed.ncbi.nlm.nih.gov

www.scholar.google.com

www.sciencedirect.com

www.cochranelibrary.com

We used the following keywords:

*In French: Fistule artério-veineuse, Accès vasculaire, Hémodialyse, Endovasculaire, Echographie-Doppler, Ellipsys, EverlinQ, WavelinQ.

*Endo Arteriovenous Fistula, Vascular Access, Hemodialysis, Endovascular, Doppler Ultrasound, Ellipsys, EverlinQ, WavelinQ.

Selection of studies

The first step involved selecting the titles and abstracts of the articles proposed by the search engines. The second step involved examining the full text to include or exclude the study in question from our work.

1)   Inclusion criteria :

Inclusion criteria included any randomised or non-randomised study that investigated the effectiveness and/or safety of endovascular AVF creation systems for HD (Endo-AVF).

2)   Exclusion criteria :

We excluded studies with the following format: case report, case series, laboratory or animal studies and literature reviews.

Data collection

The parameters collected in the different studies were:

- Characteristics of the studies

- Patient characteristics

- Patient selection criteria

- Technical success

- Maturation (time, rate)

- Primary, secondary permeability

- Interventions (rate, nature, duration)

- Procedural complications (rate, nature)

- Duration of follow-up

Definitions (1,6)

Technical success: This is angiographic evidence of rapid flow in the AVF and the absence of extravasation of blood outside the vessels.

Procedure time: The time taken to perform the endo-VAF, i.e. the time between the initial access and the removal of the catheter.

*** Maturation time:** The time to have a brachial artery flow of 500 ml/min and a vein diameter of more than 4 mm.

***Functional vascular access:** A vascular access is considered functional when it has been successfully punctured with two needles, over a period of at least six HD sessions in a 30-day period, has delivered the blood flow prescribed at the time of HD and has provided adequate HD (at least 500 ml/min).

***Primary patency: This is** the time interval between the creation of the vascular access and the first thrombosis or procedure to maintain or restore its flow.

***Primary assisted** patency**: This is** the time interval for a patented vascular access that required subsequent intervention on the upstream, access, or downstream side of the access to improve patency until it was thrombosed.

***Secondary patency: This is** the time interval for an occluded HD access or HD access that has failed haemodynamically and/or is deemed unusable for active HD and has required subsequent intervention to restore patency until thrombosis.

***Major complication**:

A serious adverse event requiring pharmacological or surgical treatment or resulting in prolonged hospitalisation.

***Intervention-related complication:** Any medical event arising directly from the intervention or device, from the beginning of the procedure to its end.

Conflicts of interest

The authors declare that they have no conflict of interest in this work.

Results

In this review, 15 published studies were selected. The results of these studies have been summarised in the tables below. Six studies were prospective, two of which were multicentre. The studies included a simple description of EverlinQ (three studies), WavelinQ (one study) or Ellipsys (six studies), or a comparison between two methods Surgery versus device or two devices (five studies) (Table I).

The number of patients included varied from 8 to 234 in the non-comparative studies and from 70 to 214 patients in the comparative studies.

Table I: Characteristics of the studies according to the device used, the number of patients and the type of study.

Author Year	Device	Patients	Foresight	Multicentric	Comparative
Rajan (7) 2015	EverlinQ	33	YES	NO	NO
Radosa (8) 2017	EverlinQ	8	NO	NO	NO
Hull (9) 2017	Ellipsys	26	YES	NO	NO
Lok (10) 2017 (NEAT)	EverlinQ	60	YES	YES	NO
Hull (11) 2018	Ellipsys	107	YES	YES	NO
Mallios (12) 2018	Ellipsys	34	NO	NO	NO
Beathard (13) 2019	Ellipsys	105	NO	YES	NO
Berland (14) 2019	WavelinQ	32	YES	NO	NO
Hebibi (15) 2019	Ellipsys	34	NO	NO	NO
Inston (16) 2019	WavelinQ vs. surgery	70 (30/40)	NO	NO	YES
Mallios (17) 2020	Ellipsys	234	NO	NO	NO
Shahverdyan (18) 2020	Ellipsys vs. WavelinQ	100 (65/35)	YES	NO	YES
Harika (19) 2021	Ellipsys vs. surgery	214 (107/107)	NO	NO	YES
Osofsky (20) 2021	Ellipsys vs. surgery	86 (24/62)	NO	NO	YES
Shahverdyan (21) 2021	Ellipsys vs. surgery	158 (89/69)	NO	NO	YES

The patients were male in more than half of the cases except in the Hull study (9). The mean age of patients was 51 years or older in all studies. Association with other defects was reported. Diabetes was reported in 12 studies and hypertension in seven studies (Table II).

Table II: Socio-medical characteristics of patients included in the studies

Author Year	Device	Patients	Average age (years)	Men (%)	Diabetes (%)	HTA (%)	HD (%)
Rajan (7) 2015	EverlinQ	33	51	61	58	-	94
Radosa (8) 2017	EverlinQ	8	57	75	50	75	-
Hull (9) 2017	Ellipsys	26	45,5	38,4	65	92	100
Lok (10) 2017	EverlinQ	60	59,9	65	50	92	43
Hull (11) 2018	Ellipsys	107	56,7	72,9	64,5	98,1	61,7
Mallios (12) 2018	Ellipsys	34	64	66,7	63	-	69
Beathard (13) 2019	Ellipsys	105	56,2	77	-	-	-
Berland (14) 2019	WavelinQ	32	51,4	97	56,3	90	3
Hebibi (15) 2019	Ellipsys	34	62	58	38	94	-
Inston (16) 2019	WavelinQ vs. surgery	70 (30/40)	57 vs 54	83 vs 72.5	-	-	87 vs 85
Mallios (17) 2020	Ellipsys	234	64	63	55	-	54
Shahverdyan (18) 2020	Ellipsys vs. WavelinQ	100 (65 vs 35)	64,2 (63.7 vs 65)	69 (63 vs 80)	37 (34 vs 43)	-	53 (51 vs 57)
Harika (19) 2021	Ellipsys vs. surgery	214 (107 vs 107)	63.6 vs 63.5	61.7 vs 60.8	-	-	61 vs 47
Osofsky (20) 2021	Ellipsys vs. surgery	86 (24 vs 62)	56.7 vs 62.5	50 vs 52	75 vs 74	88 vs. 94	58 vs 66

| Shahverdyan (21) 2021 | Ellipsys vs. surgery | 158 (89 vs 69) | 64 vs 66 | 65 vs 51 | 36 vs 48 | - | - |

vs: versus

The anastomoses were either between the ulnar artery and vein only (four studies) or ulnar and radial (three studies) or between ARP and VPC. The distance between the artery and vein was less than or equal to 1.5 cm in the majority of studies, the diameter of the arteries and veins was greater than or equal to 2 cm. The procedure time varied from 14 to 74 minutes (Table III).

Table III: Description of procedures according to anatomical criteria and procedure time.

Author Year	Device	Anastomosis	Anatomical criteria	Procedure time (minutes)
Rajan (7) 2015	EverlinQ	a and v ularies	D a-v ≤ 2 mm; Ø a and v ≥ 2 mm	-
Radosa (8) 2017	EverlinQ	a and v ularies	Ø a and v humeral ≥ 2.5 mm; a and v ulnar // and proximal ≥ 2 cm; VPC; Ø v cephalic and basilic ≥ 2 mm	-
Hull (9) 2017	Ellipsys	ARP and mail order	Radial Ø a > 2 mm Adjacent Ø v > 2 mm; Good collateral circulation Radial D a-v ≤ 1.5 mm	18.4 min
Lok (10) 2017	EverlinQ	a and v ularies	Vascular mapping	-
Hull (11) 2018	Ellipsys	ARP and mail order	Radial Ø a and adjacent v > 2 mm; Good collateral circulation; Radial Ø a-adjacent v ≤ 1.5 mm	23.7 min
Mallios (12) 2018	Ellipsys	ARP and mail order	Ø a radial > 2 mm; Ø VPC > 3 mm; D ARP-VPC < 1.5 mm	-
Beathard (13) 2019	Ellipsys	ARP and mail order	-	-
Berland (14) 2019	WavelinQ	a v ularies a v radial	Ø a v ≥2 mm	-
Hebibi (15) 2019	Ellipsys	ARP MAIL ORDER	Ø ARP and VPC ≥ 2 mm; D ARP-VPC ≤ 1.5 mm	-
Inston (16) 2019	WavelinQ vs. surgery	a v ularies a v radial	-	-
Mallios (17) 2020	Ellipsys	ARP MAIL ORDER	Ø ARP VPC ≥ 2 mm; D ARP-VPC ≤ 1.5 mm	15 min
Shahverdyan (18) 2020	Ellipsys vs. WavelinQ	ARP VPC/ a v ularies a v radial	Ellipsys: VPC, Ø VPC > 2 mm, Ø ARP > 2 mm, D ARP-VPC ≤ 1.5 mm WavelinQ: VPC, radial or ulnar humeral Ø a and v > 2 mm, D a-v < 1 mm;	14 min vs 63 min

Harika (19) 2021	Ellipsys vs. surgery	ARP MAIL ORDER	Ellipsys: Ø ARP VPC ≥ 2 mm	-
Osofsky (20) 2021	Ellipsys vs. surgery	ARP MAIL ORDER	Ellipsys: Ø ARP VPC ≥ 2 mm, D ARP-VPC ≤ 1.5 mm	60 min vs 56 min
Shahverdyan (21) 2021	Ellipsys vs. surgery	ARP MAIL ORDER	Ellipsys: Ø ARP VPC ≥ 2 mm, D ARP-VPC ≤ 1.5 mm	14 min vs 74 min

a: artery, v: vein, vs: versus, PRA: proximal radial artery, PCV: perforating elbow vein, Ø: diameter, D: distance, min: minutes

The success of the anastomoses was variable depending on the studies and the devices used. It was over 97% for EverlinQ and 88-98% for Ellipsys. The comparison between two devices or one device versus surgery showed no significant difference between the two methods. The time to maturation varied from 30 to 63 days. It was shorter for Ellipsys (30 to 45 days). The ripening rate was acceptable and was better for Ellipsys. It was better for devices compared to surgery. Maturation rate increased with time according to the Shahverdyan study published in 2021 [21].

Table IV: Results of the procedures according to technical success, delay and maturation rate.

Author Year	Device	Technical success	Ripening time (days)	Maturation rate
Rajan (7) 2015	EverlinQ	97 %	58	96% at 3 months
Radosa (8) 2017	EverlinQ	100 %	63	-
Hull (9) 2017	Ellipsys	88 %	-	-
Lok (10) 2017	EverlinQ	98 %	-	87 %
Hull (11) 2018	Ellipsys	95 %	-	-
Mallios (12) 2018	Ellipsys	97 %	45	100 %
Beathard (13) 2019	Ellipsys	98 %	-	-
Berland (14) 2019	WavelinQ	100 %	90	91 %
Hebibi (15) 2019	Ellipsys	97 %	-	-
Inston (16) 2019	WavelinQ vs. surgery	96.7% vs. 92.6%.	-	-
Mallios (17) 2020	Ellipsys	99 %	30 days	-
Shahverdyan (18) 2020	Ellipsys vs. WavelinQ	100% vs. 97%.	30 days	68.3% vs 54.3%
Harika (19) 2021	Ellipsys vs. surgery	-	45 days	65% vs. 50%.
Osofsky (20) 2021	Ellipsys vs. surgery	96% vs. 100%.		

| Shahverdyan (21) 2021 | Ellipsys vs. surgery | 100% vs. 100%. | - | | 76.4% vs 76.1% at 1 month
80.9% vs 79.1% at 3 months
85.4% vs 79.1% at 6 months |

vs: versus

The time to market varied according to the device. It ranged from 32 days for EverlinQ to 118 days for Ellipsys. The evaluation of the exploitation rate was done at intervals ranging from one to six months. It was variable within the same device and between devices. The primary patency rate was assessed at 3, 6, 12, 18 and 24 months depending on the study. It decreased with time. There was variability in the primary patency rate between studies and methods (Table V).

Table V: Results of the procedures according to time and exploitation rate and primary permeability rate

Author Year	Device	Operating time	Operating rate	Primary permeability rate
Rajan (7) 2015	EverlinQ	-	96% at 1 month	96% at 6 months
Radosa (8) 2017	EverlinQ	-	86% at 3 months	100% at 6 months
Hull (9) 2017	Ellipsys	-	80% at 1 month 70% at 3 months 60% at 6 months	87% at 6 weeks
Lok (10) 2017	EverlinQ	32 days	64 %	69% at 12 months
Hull (11) 2018	Ellipsys	118 days	88 %	98.4% at 3 months 98.4% at 6 months 92.3% at 12 months
Mallios (12) 2018	Ellipsys	45 days	100 %	94% (permeability at last check)
Beathard (13) 2019	Ellipsys	-	-	Cumulative permeability 97.1% at 6 months, 93.9% at 12 months 93.9% at 18 months, 92.7% at 24 months

Berland (14) 2019	Wavelin Q	43 days	78% at 3 months	83% at 6 months
Hebibi (15) 2019	Ellipsys	-	82% from 10 days to 6 weeks	-
Inston (16) 2019	Wavelin Q vs. surgery	130 vs 118 days	-	65.5% vs 53.4% at 6 months 56.6% vs 44% at 12 months
Mallios (17) 2020	Ellipsys	Puncture <2 weeks 10	-	54% at 1 year (primary assisted 85%)
Shahverdyan (18) 2020	Ellipsys vs. Wavelin Q	60 vs 90 days	79.5% vs. 58%. 5 vs 1 puncture on day 1 er	33% vs 32% at 1 year
Harika (19) 2021	Ellipsys vs. surgery	-	61% vs. 47%.	61% vs 86% at 1 year 55% vs 52% at 2 years
Osofsky (20) 2021	Ellipsys vs. surgery	-	53% vs. 87%.	-
Shahverdyan (21) 2021	Ellipsys vs. surgery	57 vs 68 days	84.5% vs. 79.4%.	61% vs 64% at 1 year

vs: versus

The secondary patency rate was satisfactory (above 75%) regardless of the procedure. It decreased slightly with time (Table VI).

Table VI: Procedural outcomes by procedure and secondary patency rate

Author Year	Device	Intervention rates	Interventions	Secondary permeability rate
Rajan (7) 2015	Everlin Q	0.6/patient	V brachial embolisation; Surgical AVF; Thrombin injection; Cephalic TAA; Central TAA	75 %
Radosa (8) 2017	Everlin Q	0 %	-	-
Hull (9) 2017	Ellipsys	87 %	TKA 43%; V brachial embolization 26%; Basilic ligation 17%; Transposition 30%; Valvulotomy 4%.	-
Lok (10) 2017	Everlin Q	0.46/patient/year	5 basilic transpositions; 5 v brachial embolizations; 3 ligations; 2 thrombin injections; 2 LTAs; 1 thrombolysis, 2 thrombectomies; 2 surgical repairs; 2 new AVFs or bypasses	84% (cumulative)

Hull (11) 2018	Ellipsys	2.7/patient/year (271)	Maturation (205) : ATL anastomosis; Basilic v brachial embolization; Transposition Maintenance (66) : ATL; Embolisation; Stent	91.6% at 3 months 89.3% at 6 months 86.7% at 1 year (cumulative)
Mallios (12) 2018	Ellipsys	0 %	-	-
Beathard (13) 2019	Ellipsys	-	-	-
Berland (14) 2019	Wavelin Q	0.21/patient/year	ATL	87% (cumulative)
Hebibi (15) 2019	Ellipsys	35 %	ATL; Basilicar median banding; Valvulotomy; Surgical AVF	-
Inston (16) 2019	Wavelin Q vs. surgery	0.4 vs 0.27/patient/year	ATL; Stent; Coil embolisation; Transposition/Revision; Thrombolysis; Thrombectomy	75.8% vs 66.7 at 6 months 69.5% vs 57.6% at 12 months
Mallios (17) 2020	Ellipsys	-	Surgical conversion 1%; Superficialisation 10%;	96% at 1 year
Shahverdyan (18) 2020	Ellipsys vs. Wavelin Q	27.7% vs. 26.5%. 0.96 vs 0.46/patient/year	-	82% vs 60% at 1 year
Harika (19) 2021	Ellipsys vs. surgery	53% vs 36% at 1 year 70% vs 79% at 2 years	at 1 year: Percutaneous: 41% vs 4%; Surgical: 12% vs 33%. at 2 years: Percutaneous: 53% vs 42%; Surgical: 17% vs 36%.	91% vs 90% at 1 year 91% vs 88% at 2 years
Osofsky (20) 2021	Ellipsys vs. surgery	1.1 vs 0.3/patient/year 57% vs. 8%. 9% vs. 3%. 4% vs. 3%. 3% vs. 13%.	ATL Cephalic or basilic coil embolisation Ligation of the cephalic or basilic v Superficialisation or transposition of the cephalic or basilica	-
Shahverdyan (21) 2021	Ellipsys vs. surgery	1 patient vs 0	Surgical conversion	34% vs 12% at 1 year

AVF: arteriovenous fistula, TLA: transluminal angioplasty, ve: vein, vs: versus,

The total follow-up time varied from 6 months to 2 years. The rate of major complications was variable. With advances in device technology, the major complication rate has been reduced, resulting in improved fistula patency (Table VII).

Table VII: Outcomes of procedures according to complications

Author Year	Device	Major complication rate	Complications	Total follow-up time
Rajan (7) 2015	EverlinQ	3 %	Pseudo aneurysm; Thrombosis	6 months
Radosa (8) 2017	EverlinQ	0 %	-	6 months
Hull (9) 2017	Ellipsys	0 %	-	1 year
Lok (10) 2017	EverlinQ	5 %	Loss of access	1 year

Hull (11) 2018	Ellipsys	0%	-	1 year
Mallios (12) 2018	Ellipsys	0	-	141 days
Beathard (13) 2019	Ellipsys	-	-	2 years
Berland (14) 2019	WavelinQ	3 %	Loss of access	6 months
Hebibi (15) 2019	Ellipsys	2 patients	Difficulty of punctures→ surgical conversion	14 months
Inston (16) 2019	WavelinQ vs. surgery	0 %	-	1 year
Mallios (17) 2020	Ellipsys	0 %	-	302 days
Shahverdyan (18) 2020	Ellipsys vs. WavelinQ	15.4% vs. 37.1%.	Loss of access	183 vs 185 days
Harika (19) 2021	Ellipsys vs. surgery	0.9% vs. 9 0 patients vs 3 0 patients vs 4	Infection and delayed healing Aneurysm Ischemic flight syndrome	2 years
Osofsky (20) 2021	Ellipsys vs. surgery	4% vs. 0%. 0% vs. 3%. 4% vs. 0%. 4% vs. 2%. 0% vs. 3%. 0% vs. 2%. 0% vs. 2%.	30-day mortality Hematoma Oedema Pain on puncture Ischemic flight syndrome Post-operative bleeding Surgical site infection	6.1 months vs. 2.7 months
Shahverdyan (21) 2021	Ellipsys vs. surgery	1 patient vs 0	False anastomotic aneurysm→ surgical conversion	226 days vs 472 days

vs: versus,

Discussion

Native AVFs are widely regarded as the most effective access for HD in patients with CKD. Since the introduction of surgical AVF by Brescia et al (22)various surgical AVF techniques have been developed. However, these fistulas remain at high risk of maturation failure and acute thrombosis (23,24). Multiple interventions may also be required to support and maintain fistula patency and function. (25).

In a meta-analysis with systematic review of the literature that examined the efficacy and safety of endovascular AVF creation systems, Wee et al. demonstrated that technical success, maturation and short-term patency rates are acceptable, with a low risk of procedure-related complications (6). The results of our study are consistent with these findings. To our knowledge, this is the most recent review of the literature.

Endovascular AVF creation is an interesting alternative in the management of patients with ESRD. Indeed, these techniques have considerable advantages. It avoids the need for surgery and reduces AVF flow by implanting the device in the radial or ulnar artery rather than the brachial artery. It should be noted that there is insufficient experience to evaluate these techniques in the long term.

However, these techniques have their drawbacks. These include the difficulty of predicting venous drainage in the superficial and deep networks. This unpredictable incident often requires a surgical revision. Another element is the high initial cost of the devices. The data are still considered insufficient for reimbursement of these devices in France. In any case, they cannot currently replace the creation of an AVF at the wrist in the first instance when the conditions for this are met (3).

Reminder of the vascular anatomy of the elbow fold

Techniques for creating AVF percutaneously primarily use the elbow crease area. Devices are developed to create communication between an adjacent artery and vein. This anatomical configuration is uncommon in the human body, especially in vessel sizes that are reasonably accessible to endovascular punctures and tools. However, the elbow crease and the origin of the forearm arteries represent a prime site for this (Figure 1).

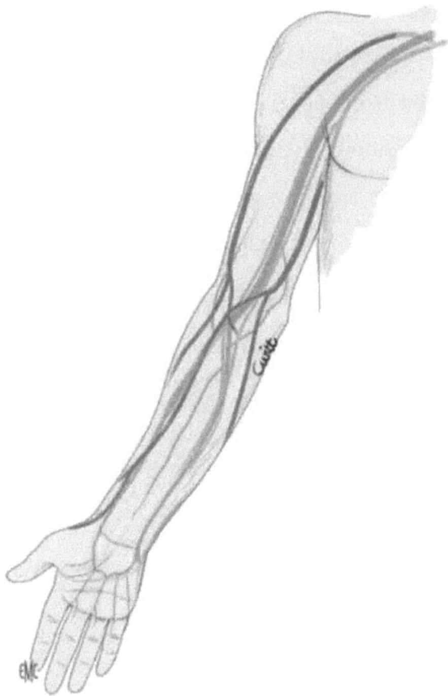

Figure 1: Vascular anatomy of the upper limb (3)

The brachial artery is located at the medial bicipital groove in the brachial canal. Behind the aponeurotic extension of the biceps muscle, it divides into a radial artery, medial to the brachioradialis muscle, and an ulnar artery, which branches off at right angles, obliquely downwards and medially, to run behind the arch of the superficial flexor muscle of the fingers. The radial artery gives the anterior radial recurrent artery which ascends into the lateral bicipital groove, while the ulnar artery gives the trunk of the interosseous arteries and the ulnar recurrent arteries (Figure 1).

Deep veins, often double, travel with their respective arteries. The superficial venous network forms the letter "M", with three superficial veins of the forearm: the cephalic vein of **the** forearm (comes from the thumb), the basilic vein of the forearm and the median vein of the forearm. These three veins join together into two trunks: the cephalic vein of the arm externally and the basilic vein of the arm medially (Figure 1). Numerous variants are described, but in three quarters of cases there is a perforating vein, called the communicating vein or elbow perforator, which connects the superficial and deep venous networks at the elbow. This vein can be used to create AVFs (3).

How does the creation of an endovascular AVF proceed?

1) Ellipsys system :

The Ellipsys® Vascular Access System (Avenu Medical, San Juan Capistrano, California, USA) is a single catheter system (Figure 2). It is used to create a percutaneous vascular anastomosis between adjacent blood vessels. It relies on direct current thermal heating to fuse the arterial and venous wall. This creates an anastomosis between the PRA and PCV in the antecubital fossa where the two anatomical elements are adjacent to each other (12).

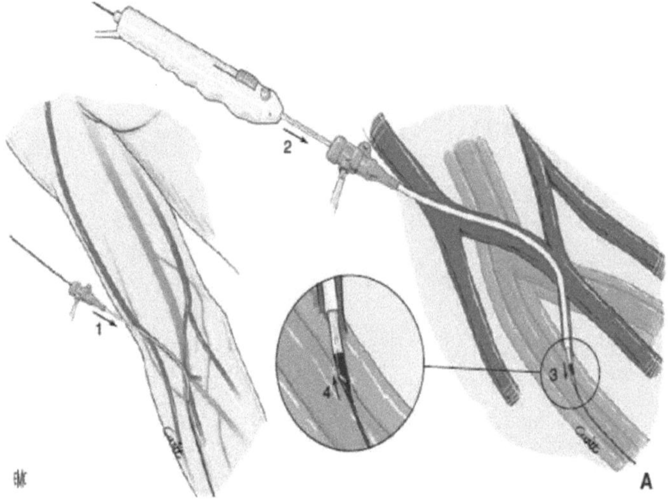

Figure 2: Percutaneous arteriovenous fistula creation, Ellipsys®
device (4)

*The cephalic vein is punctured under ultrasound control, then the needle is
advanced to the PCV and from there to the PRA. A guidewire is inserted (1),
followed by an introducer and the Ellipsys® device (2). The device is placed at the
fistula site (3), so that pressure can be applied between artery and vein and a burn
is generated by the external generator (4).

The procedure is entirely ultrasound-guided. Under locoregional anaesthesia (axillary block). It involves ultrasound-guided puncture of the medial cephalic or basilic vein in the arm retrogradely with a 22G micropuncture needle, progressing with a 0.014" guide to the PCV where it is adjacent to the radial artery, and puncturing the radial artery through this adjacent vein (9). A 0.021" guidewire is then positioned in the SVC, followed by a 6F introducer which is advanced into the SVC where it is adjacent to the radial artery (Figure 2).

The micropuncture needle is advanced over the guidewire to the same position in the vein. Under continuous ultrasound visualization of the needle tip, a puncture of the PRA is performed, creating a fistula between the PCV and the PRA. The guidewire is advanced into the radial artery. The position is checked under ultrasound guidance. A 0.014" guidewire (replacing the 0.021" guidewire) and a 6F introducer are then placed in the PRA. Then the Ellipsys® device (which is a single catheter system) is inserted through the introducer (Figure 2). It uses thermal energy to create the anastomosis between the two vessels in a matter of seconds by tissue fusion (burn-weld). Immediate dilation of the anastomosis with a 5 x 20 mm balloon accelerates maturation of the AVF. This technique, performed under ultrasound guidance, has the advantage of avoiding the use of contrast products and exposure to ionising radiation (11,12).

2) EverlinQ/WavelinQ System:

The WavelinQ™ EndoAVF System (Becton Dickinson Medical, Franklin Lakes, New Jersey, USA; formerly EverlinQ™ , TVA Medical Inc, Austin, Texas, USA) is a dual catheter system (one venous and one arterial) that uses RF energy. This creates an arteriovenous anastomosis between the arteries and deep veins of the proximal forearm, the ulnar artery and its satellite vein or the radial artery and its satellite vein (Figure 3). The superficial veins then receive arterialised blood flow via the PCV (26).

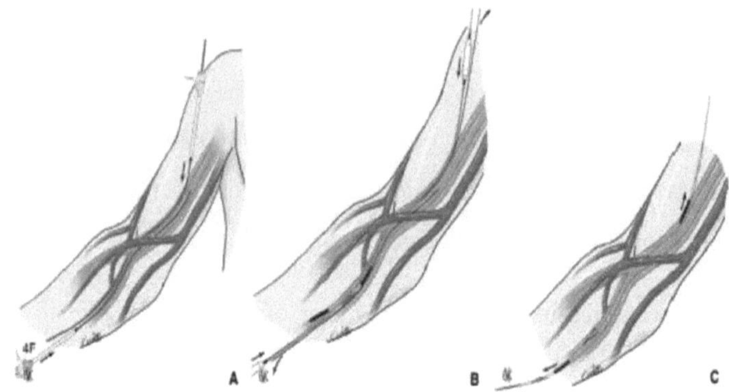

Figure 3: Percutaneous arteriovenous fistula creation, WavelinQ®
device (3)

A: Vein and artery are punctured under ultrasound control and two introducers are placed; **B:** The two WavelinQ catheters are inserted and advanced to the segment chosen for the creation of the AVF, here between the ulnar artery and the satellite ulnar vein, close to the PCV. The two catheters are magnetised and face each other. The external generator is operated, creating a radiofrequency burn at the chosen segment; **C:** the fistula thus created, the devices are removed.

The first generation EverlinQ system had a 6F diameter and required puncture of the humeral artery and vein. The second generation system now has a reduced diameter of 4F WavelinQ. Puncture can be performed at the radial artery and vein or ulnar artery and vein if anatomy permits (26). Under local anaesthesia (axillary block), a vein and an artery are punctured (using 21G micropuncture needles) (Figure 3). Subsequently, the anterograde or retrograde progression of two catheters (one arterial and one venous) results in the creation of an AVF between the proximal ulnar (or radial) artery and the ulnar (or radial) vein satellite to the artery (14).

Punctures can be made in the wrist or arm (sometimes both). They can be ultrasound-guided, but the progression and creation of the AVF is done under scopy. The two catheters are aligned opposite each other at the desired site using magnets. The AVF itself is created using an RF probe (Figure 3). The authors recommend almost systematic embolisation of at least one brachial vein to force the flow of the AVF into the superficial network, thus contributing to the maturation of the AVF. This procedure requires only an antecubital fossa and forearm angiogram at the beginning of the procedure, which reduces the volume of contrast medium required (7,8,10).

Endovascular AVF or surgical AVF?

There are multiple puncture sites and vessels that can be modified by conventional or endovascular means. They allow the choice of AVF creation to be optimised (Figure 4).

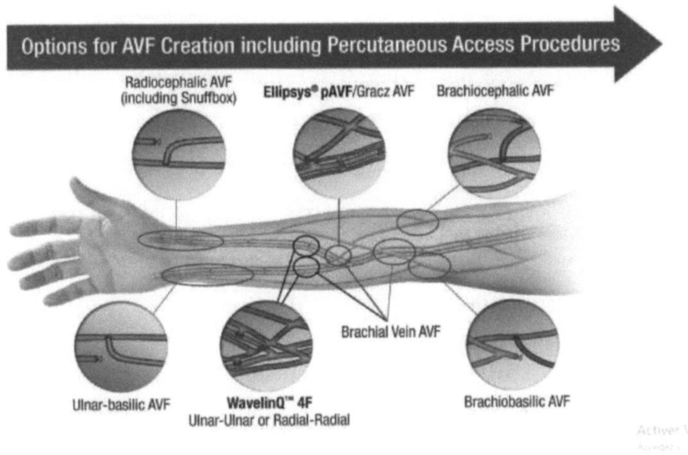

Figure 4: Endo AVF creation sites in the proximal forearm (18)

Inston et al. (16) conducted a retrospective comparative study, using a prospectively collected database between 2016 and 2019, with the objective of comparing two matched groups of endovascular AVFs created by the WavelinQ device (30 cases) to surgical radio-cephalic AVFs (40 cases). Procedural success was high, with 96.7% for the endovascular group and 92.6% for the surgical group.

Primary patency at six and 12 months was higher in the endovascular group (65.5% at six months and 56.5% at 12 months versus 53.4% and 44%). Secondary patency at six and 12 months was higher in the endovascular group (75.8% at six months and 69.5% at 12 months versus 66.7% and 57.6%). The authors concluded that endovascular AVFs created by the WavelinQ device could be considered as a first option in creating blood access, especially if the vessels in the wrist are absent or not of the right calibre to create a surgical AVF.

Harika et al. (19) conducted a single-centre retrospective comparative study of 107 patients who had an AVF created with the Ellipsys system between May 2017 and May 2018 with an equal number of patients who had a vascular access created at the same centre during the same period. The aim was to compare the outcomes of percutaneous AVFs created with the Ellipsys device and surgical AVFs. Endovascular AVFs had higher rates of maturation at six weeks (65% versus 50%). Primary patency rates were higher for surgical AVFs at 12 months (86% vs 61%). However, primary patency was similar between the two groups at 24 months (52% vs 55%). There was no significant difference in secondary patency rates at 12 (90% vs 91%) or 24 months (88% vs 91%).

After two years of follow-up, the rate of endovascular interventions was similar but surgical AVFs required more frequent surgical revisions (36% vs 17%). Wound healing and infection problems were more common in surgical AVFs (9% vs. 0.9%). Percutaneously created AVFs with the Ellipsys device had higher maturation rates and similar patency to surgical AVFs created in an experienced high volume vascular surgery department. Endovascular AVFs had a lower risk of healing problems, infection and revision surgery (19). However, larger prospective randomised multicentre studies are needed to confirm these results.

A single-centre retrospective study was performed by Osofky et al. (20) comparing the outcomes of endovascular AVFs created with the Ellipsys system from January 1, 2019 to December 31, 2019 (24 cases) with those of humerocephalic surgical AVFs created from January 1, 2018 to December 31, 2018 (62 cases). The endovascular and surgical AVF groups had comparable mean procedure times (60 vs 56 min) and technical success rates (96% vs 100%). The endovascular group had a lower maturation rate (52% vs 87%) and a higher primary failure rate compared to the surgical group (39% vs 10%).

The endovascular group had a higher rate of postoperative interventions (78% versus 21%), as well as a higher total number of postoperative interventions (1.1 versus 0.3). Percutaneous juxta-anastomotic transluminal angioplasty was the most frequent postoperative procedure in the endovascular group and occurred at a significantly higher frequency (57% versus 8%). The authors concluded that patients with endovascular AVF using the Ellipsys system had lower rates of maturation and more postoperative procedures compared to patients with surgically created humerocephalic AVF (20). The discrepancies in results compared to previously reported Ellipsys data highlighted the need for further studies examining the feasibility of endovascular AVFs with these endovascular devices.

Shahverdyan et al. (21) conducted a retrospective study of prospectively collected clinical data comparing the outcomes of endovascular AVF (89 cases) created by the Ellipsys device with those of surgical AVF of the proximal forearm (69 cases). Patients were enrolled over a 34-month period. Technical success was 100% for both groups. The average procedure time was 14 minutes for percutaneous AVFs and 74 minutes for surgical AVFs. PRA was used in all cases of endovascular AVF. Radial (30%), ulnar (12%) and brachial (58%) arteries were used for surgical AVF. The drainage veins for both groups were cephalic and/or basilic veins.

AVF flow rate, maturation time and number of procedures per patient year were not significantly different. The cumulative incidence of primary patency failure at 12 months was lower for surgical AVFs (47% vs. 64%), but secondary patency failure did not differ between groups (20% vs. 12%). Endovascular and surgical AVFs had similar primary patency (65% vs 64%). Secondary patency failure rates were higher for surgical AVFs than endovascular AVFs (34% vs. 12%) at 12 months (21).

The authors concluded that both endovascular and surgical AVFs demonstrated high rates of technical success and secondary patency. Endovascular AVFs had shorter procedure times. The intervention rate was similar. When a distal radial AVF is not feasible, percutaneous AVF may be an appropriate procedure to create safe and functional access, leaving other options for creating surgical AVFs in the proximal forearm (21).

What is the cost of endovascular AVFs?

Due to the early and late failures that can occur with surgically created AVFs, re-interventions are often required to facilitate AVF maturation and maintain patency. A study was conducted to compare re-interventions and their associated costs in patients with surgically created AVFs and those with endovascularly created AVFs using the EverlinQ device in the NEAT Trial (27). Of the 3764 patients with surgical AVFs created from 2011 to 2013 from Medicare (Medicare Standard Analytical Files), 60 were successfully matched to patients with surgical AVFs.

The rate of re-interventions within one year was lower for patients with endovascular AVFs (0.59 per patient/year) compared with the matched surgical AVF group (3.43 per patient/year). For the endovascular AVF group, the rate of angioplasty, thrombectomy, catheter placement, subsequent arteriovenous bypass surgery, new surgical AVF, and access-related infection were significantly lower in the endovascular AVF group than in the surgical AVF group. The average first year cost per patient year associated with post-creation procedures was estimated to be less than US$11,240 for endovascular AVF compared to surgical AVF. (27).

A literature review was conducted by Rognoni et al. (28) to perform cost-effectiveness and budget impact analyses comparing the creation of endovascular AVFs with the creation of surgical AVFs in haemodialysis patients at the National Healthcare Service in Italy. The authors concluded that endovascular AVFs created by the WavelinQ device were associated with lower cost and better quality of life for patients. The gradual increase in WavelinQ device usage rates compared to surgical AVFs over five years is expected to save the National Healthcare Service in Italy an estimated €30-36 million overall.

Ellipsys system or WavelinQ system?

Shahverdyan et al. (18) conducted a single-centre retrospective study between December 2017 and December 2019 to compare the clinical outcomes of AVFs created by the Ellipsys and WavelinQ systems. 100 patients (65 Ellipsys; 35 WavelinQ) were included, 69% of whom were male, 37% of whom had diabetes. The average age was 64 years. The results of Ellipsys were compared with those of WavelinQ. The technical success was 100% versus 97% respectively. The average procedure time was 14 versus 63 minutes, with an equal average follow-up (183 versus 185 days). Maturation at four weeks was 68.3% versus 54.3%. The average time to puncture was 60 versus 90 days. A successful HD session was achieved with endovascular AVFs in 31 of 39 patients (79.5%) versus 14 of 24 patients (58%).

Access-related adverse events were observed in four patients (1 Ellipsys versus 3 WavelinQ). Interventions were performed in 27.7% (33 Ellipsys) and 26.5% (15 WavelinQ) of patients. The number of interventions per patient/year was 0.96 versus 0.46. Endovascular AVF failure was observed in 15.4% versus 37.1% of patients, respectively. Secondary patency at 12 months was significantly higher in patients who underwent the Ellipsys procedure (82%) than in those who underwent the WavelinQ procedure (60%). The authors concluded that endovascular AVFs were created with high technical success with few complications with both devices. However, the Ellipsys system had significantly shorter procedure times, no exposure to ionising radiation and superior secondary patency.

The results of our study should be interpreted with caution as the majority of studies are retrospective and all non-randomised. They are therefore subject to selection bias and confounding bias. In addition, there is a lack of long-term data due to the short follow-up time in some studies. Larger multi-centre studies with a larger number of patients and a longer post-operative follow-up time are needed comparing the results of endovascular AVFs with those of surgical AVFs. These studies would help determine the place of endovascular AVFs in the management of patients with ESRD.

Conclusions

It is accepted nowadays that native AVF is the best vascular approach for HD. Recently, new minimally invasive techniques for endovascular AVF fabrication have emerged: the Ellipsys® system and the WavelinQ™ system.

In this work, we conducted a literature review to assess the efficacy and safety of endo-VAF creation systems in patients with ESRD. The review included 15 publications with the inclusion criteria being any randomised or non-randomised study that investigated the efficacy and safety of endo-VAF creation systems; and the exclusion criteria being any study in the format of a case report, case series, laboratory or animal studies, and reviews of the literature.

Four studies were prospective and multicentre, five studies were comparative and none were randomised. The total number of patients was 1301. Only one study compared the Ellipsys/WavelinQ systems, the other four studies compared endo-VAF devices to surgery. Five studies evaluated the EverlinQ / WavelinQ system.

The overall technical success rate for all endo-VAF systems was 96.5%. For the EverlinQ / WavelinQ systems the rate was 96.5%. For the Ellipsys system, the success rate was 96.6%. The overall maturation rate at 3 months for all endo-VAF systems combined was 80.2%. For the EverlinQ / WavelinQ systems, this rate was 81.85% and 79.55% for the Ellipsys system.

The overall primary patency rate of the endo-AVFs was 89.6% at 6 months and 61.7% at 12 months. The primary patency rate for the EverlinQ / WavelinQ systems was 86% at 6 months and 52.5% at 12 months. The primary patency rate for the Ellipsys system was 94% at 6 months and 66% at 12 months.

The overall complication rate for all endo-VAF systems was 10.4%. For the EverlinQ / WavelinQ systems, the rate was 12%. For the Ellipsys system, it was 8.7%. The average follow-up time for patients was 323.8 days.

The advantage of endo-AVFs is that they avoid surgical approach and limit AVF flow by implanting in the distal radial or ulnar artery (not the humeral one); thus minimising complications such as ischaemic steal syndrome.

On the other hand, endo-VAFs have certain disadvantages, which are their high cost and the difficult-to-predict venous drainage, both in the superficial and deep network, often requiring re-intervention (embolisation by co-injection of the humeral vein for the EverlinQ / WavelinQ systems), thus increasing the costs of the interventions.

In the absence of sufficient hindsight, data are still considered insufficient to judge the superiority of these minimally invasive procedures over conventional surgery. Endo-VAF could not replace, at present, surgical AVF performed in first intention at the wrist when the anatomical conditions are met for it.

The results of our study should be interpreted with caution as the majority of studies are retrospective and are all non-randomised. They are therefore subject to selection bias and confounding bias. Furthermore, there is a lack of long-term data due to the novelty of these procedures and the short duration of follow-up.

Larger-scale, prospective, randomised, multicentre studies with long post-operative follow-up are needed to compare the outcomes of endo-AVFs with those of surgical AVFs; to determine their place in the management of patients with ESRD. Given the global CKD epidemic and limited health budgets, it is still reasonable to be cautious about the primary indication for these expensive medical devices.

Given the satisfactory efficacy and safety of the current endovascular AVF systems, they could be an alternative for patients with eligibility criteria. However, at present they should not be considered as a first line solution and their superiority cannot be confirmed due to the lack of prospective, comparative, multicentre, randomised studies comparing surgical and endovascular AVF creation with long postoperative follow-up

With the epidemic of kidney failure worldwide, and limited health budgets, it is reasonable to be cautious about the use of expensive medical devices. It seems clear that endovascular AVF creation will become the gold standard for CKD patients. As technology advances, the technique is refined and the experience of the teams improves, the results will continue to improve.

References

1.   Schmidli J, Widmer MK, Basile C, de Donato G, Gallieni M, Gibbons CP, et al. Editor's Choice - Vascular Access: 2018 Clinical Practice Guidelines of the European Society for Vascular Surgery (ESVS). Eur J Vasc Endovasc Surg. 2018;55(6):757-818.

2.   Committee I, Editors MJ. HD Medical Press. 2004;89(3):264.

3.   Sadaghianloo N, Declemy S. Creation of vascular outlets for haemodialysis: strategy and operative techniques. Encycl Med Chir (Elsevier Masson, Paris), Vascular Surgery, 43-029-R, 2020, 15p.

4.   Marzelle J, Bourquelot P. Hemodialysis vascular approaches (continued): arteriovenous bypass, central venous catheters, overall strategy. Encycl Med Chir (Elsevier Masson, Paris), Chirurgie vasculaire, 43-029-S, 2014, 10p.

5.   Mallios A, Houérou TLE, Harika G, Canonge J, Blic RDE, Costanzo A, et al. Percutaneous arteriovenous fistula creation for hemodialysis. 2019;1-6.

6.   Yan Wee IJ, Yap HY, Tang TY, Chong TT. A systematic review, meta-analysis, and meta-regression of the efficacy and safety of endovascular arteriovenous fistula creation. J Vasc Surg [Internet]. 2020;71(1):309-317.c5. Available from: https://doi.org/10.1016/j.jvs.2019.07.057

7.   Rajan DK, Ebner A, Desai SB, Rios JM, Cohn WE. Percutaneous creation of an arteriovenous fistula for hemodialysis access. J Vasc Interv Radiol [Internet]. 2015;26(4):484-90. Available from: http://dx.doi.org/10.1016/j.jvir.2014.12.018

8.   Radosa CG, Radosa JC, Weiss N, Schmidt C, Werth S, Hofmockel T, et al. Endovascular Creation of an Arteriovenous Fistula (endoAVF) for Hemodialysis Access: First Results. Cardiovasc Intervent Radiol. 2017;40(10):1545-51.

9.   Hull JE, Elizondo-riojas G, Bishop W, Voneida-reyna YL. Thermal Resistance Anastomosis Device for the Percutaneous Creation of Arteriovenous Fistulae for Hemodialysis. J Vasc Interv Radiol [Internet]. 2017;(5):1-8. Available from: http://dx.doi.org/10.1016/j.jvir.2016.10.033

10. Lok C, Rajan DK, Clement J, Kiaii M, Sidhu R, Thomson K, et al. Endovascular Proximal Forearm Arteriovenous Fistula for Hemodialysis Access: Results of the Prospective, Multicenter Novel Endovascular Access Trial (NEAT). Am J Kidney Dis. 2017;70(4):486-97.

11. Hull JE, Jennings WC, Cooper RI, Waheed U, Schaefer ME, Narayan R. The Pivotal Multicenter Trial of Ultrasound-Guided Percutaneous Arteriovenous Fistula Creation for Hemodialysis Access. J Vasc Interv Radiol [Internet]. 2018;29(2):149-158.e5. Available from: https://doi.org/10.1016/j.jvir.2017.10.015

12. Mallios A, Jennings WC, Boura B, Costanzo A, Bourquelot P, Combes M. Early results of percutaneous arteriovenous fistula creation with the

Ellipsys Vascular Access System. J Vasc Surg [Internet]. 2018;68(4):1150-6. Available from: https://doi.org/10.1016/j.jvs.2018.01.036

13. Beathard GA, Litchfield T, Jennings WC. Two-year cumulative patency of endovascular arteriovenous fistula. J Vasc Access. 2019;21(3):350-6.

14. Berland TL, Clement J, Griffin J, Westin GG, Ebner A. Endovascular Creation of Arteriovenous Fistulae for Hemodialysis Access with a 4 Fr Device: Clinical Experience from the EASE Study. Ann Vasc Surg [Internet]. 2019;60:182-92. Available from: https://doi.org/10.1016/j.avsg.2019.02.023

15. Hebibi H, Achiche J, Franco G, Rottembourg J. Clinical hemodialysis experience with percutaneous arteriovenous fistulas created using the Ellipsys® vascular access system. Hemodial Int. 2019;23(2):167-72.

16. Inston N, Khawaja A, Tullett K, Jones R. WavelinQ created arteriovenous fistulas versus surgical radiocephalic observational study. 2019;

17. Mallios A, Bourquelot P, Franco G, Hebibi H. Midterm results of percutaneous arteriovenous fi stula creation with the Ellipsys Vascular Access System , technical recommendations , and an algorithm for maintenance. J Vasc Surg [Internet]. 2020;1-10. Available from: https://doi.org/10.1016/j.jvs.2020.02.048

18. Shahverdyan R, Beathard G, Mushtaq N, Litch TF, Nelson PR, Jennings WC. Comparison of Outcomes of Percutaneous Arteriovenous Fistulae Creation by Ellipsys and WavelinQ Devices. 2020;1365-72.

19. Harika G, Mallios A, Allouache M, Costanzo A, de Blic R, Boura B, et al. Comparison of surgical versus percutaneously created arteriovenous hemodialysis fistulae. J Vasc Surg [Internet]. 2021; Available from: https://doi.org/10.1016/j.jvs.2020.12.086

20. Osofsky R, Byrd D, Reagor J, Das Gupta J, Clark R, Argyropoulos C, et al. Initial Outcomes Following Introduction of Percutaneous Arteriovenous Fistula Program with Comparison to Historical Surgically Created Fistulas. Ann Vasc Surg [Internet]. 2021; Available from: https://doi.org/10.1016/j.avsg.2020.12.041

21. Shahverdyan R, Beathard G, Mushtaq N, Litchfield TF, Vartanian S, Konner K, et al. Comparison of Ellipsys Percutaneous and Proximal Forearm Gracz-Type Surgical Arteriovenous Fistulas. Am J Kidney Dis [Internet]. 2021; Available from: https://doi.org/10.1053/j.ajkd.2021.01.011

22. Brescia MJ, Cimino JE, Appel K, Hurwich BJ. Chronic hemodialysis using venipuncture and a surgically created arteriovenous fistula. New Engl J Med. 1966;275(20):1089-966.

23. Al-Jaishi AA, Oliver MJ, Thomas SM, Lok CE, Zhang JC, Garg AX, et al. Patency rates of the arteriovenous fistula for hemodialysis: A systematic

review and meta-analysis. Am J Kidney Dis [Internet]. 2014;63(3):464-78. Available from: http://dx.doi.org/10.1053/j.ajkd.2013.08.023

24. Falk A. Maintenance and Salvage of Arteriovenous Fistulas. 2005;807-13.

25. Biuckians A, Scott EC, Meier GH, Panneton JM, Glickman MH. The natural history of autologous fistulas as first-time dialysis access in the KDOQI era. 2009;415-21.

26. Dawoud D, Lok CE, Waheed U. Recent Advances in Arteriovenous Access Creation for Hemodialysis: New Horizons in Dialysis Vascular Access. Adv Chronic Kidney Dis [Internet]. 2020;27(3):191-8. Available from: https://doi.org/10.1053/j.ackd.2020.02.002

27. Yang S, Lok C, Arnold R, Rajan D, Glickman M. Comparison of post-creation procedures and costs between surgical and an endovascular approach to arteriovenous fistula creation. J Vasc Access. 2017;18(Suppl 2):s8-14.

28. Rognoni C, Tozzi M, Tarricone R. Endovascular versus surgical creation of arteriovenous fistula in hemodialysis patients: Cost-effectiveness and budget impact analyses. J Vasc Access. 2020;

Summary

Native AVF is considered the best vascular approach. Surgical arteriovenous fistulas (AVFs) were first described over 50 years ago and have revolutionised the outlook for millions of dialysis-dependent patients. Despite numerous developments, outcomes are sub-optimal, with high rates of primary failure and re-intervention to maintain patency. Surgical AVFs are known to fail in part because of intimal hyperplasia leading to stenosis and manipulation of the vessel during creation of the anastomosis may contribute to this.

Recently, new minimally invasive techniques for endovascular AVF fabrication have emerged: the Ellipsys® system and the WavelinQ™ system. These new technologies allow the creation of AVFs for HD endovascularly with minimal trauma to the vessel. In this literature review, we present the place of endovascular AVFs in the management of haemodialysis patients, patient selection criteria, trial results, technical aspects, reinterventions and future prospects.

The results are encouraging, with high technical success rates and low re-intervention and failure rates. The results of our study should be interpreted with caution as the majority of studies are retrospective and all are non-randomised. There is a lack of long-term data due to the short follow-up time in some studies.

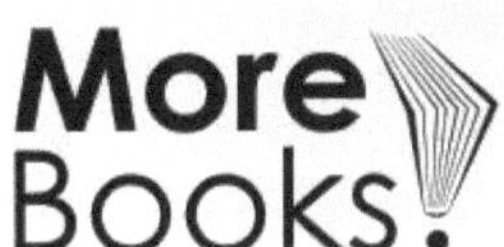

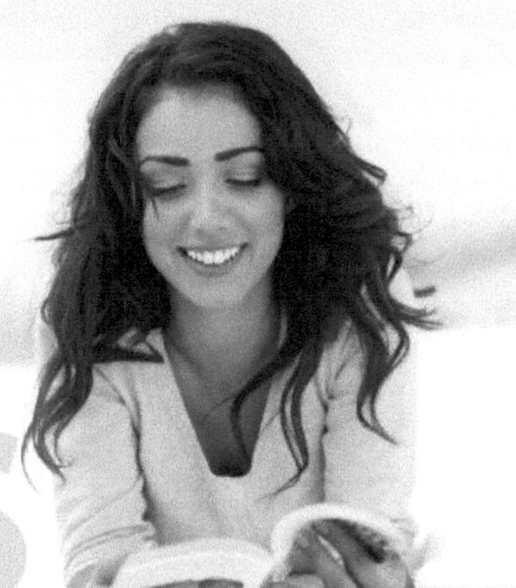

I want morebooks!

Buy your books fast and straightforward online - at one of world's fastest growing online book stores! Environmentally sound due to Print-on-Demand technologies.

Buy your books online at
www.morebooks.shop

Kaufen Sie Ihre Bücher schnell und unkompliziert online – auf einer der am schnellsten wachsenden Buchhandelsplattformen weltweit! Dank Print-On-Demand umwelt- und ressourcenschonend produzi ert.

Bücher schneller online kaufen
www.morebooks.shop

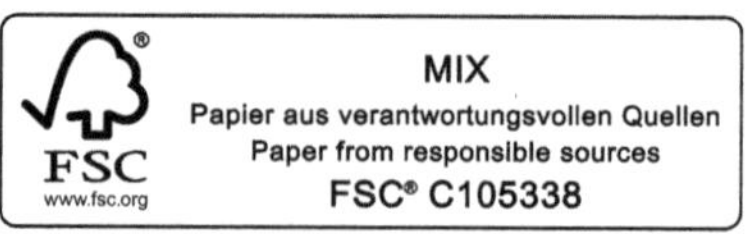

Printed by Books on Demand GmbH, Norderstedt / Germany